Table of Contents

The Potential Link Between Nose Picking and Alzheimer's Disease: A Comprehensive Review

The Potential Link Between Nose Picking and Alzheimer's

1. Introduction to Nose Picking and Alzheimer's

However, most of the time, nose picking is not harmful. And guess what? While doctors and scientists are doing a lot of research on Alzheimer's, no one has ever thought about examining the potential link between picking your nose and the development of Alzheimer's disease. In simpler terms, clicking on the title of that 'article' would lead to a publication titled 'April Fools', detailing why people fall for hoaxes and fake news on the internet on April 1 every year. In short, there is no reason to believe nose picking and the chances of developing Alzheimer's are linked in any way. If you were looking forward to some exciting research into the habit, we're afraid we have some bad news.

An article has been circulating on social media that draws a potential link between nose picking and Alzheimer's. The claim has received negative feedback for not being backed up. However, picking our nose is generally considered an unhygienic habit. Our noses produce mucus throughout the day, and that mucus helps eliminate dust, dirt, and other foreign contaminants that we breathe in. We generally swallow our mucus. However, if that mucus becomes thicker for any reason, we tend to lift it up to our mouth and spit it out. This is especially true if we have a cold or allergies. Once in a while, we might pick our nose too aggressively. The blood vessels in our nose and the tissue surrounding them are quite delicate and can get damaged if the tip of our picky finger is sharp enough.

1.1. Definition and Prevalence of Nose Picking

Nose picking often results in the deposition of the excreta on surfaces that are touched by a large, if unknowable, number of individuals who have yet to wash their hands. However, some positive public attitudes towards nose excreta were found, that were the non-bose equivalent of commercial boogers. It was found that only "30% of adults pick their nose and around 60% of school-age children pick their nose regularly". A group of over 500 pregnant females were asked about nose picking and how it did or did not impress bumper stickers.

Some of the few scholars to study nose picking lend no empirical evidence of the phenomenon but are intrigued by the possible links to purified public and private minds. Writing about table manners, Rustin (1992) suggests that a foundation for discussing the potential connections between nose picking and pure (Alzheimer's) minds is the "commonplace unexamined comment that nose picking is a repugnant and disgusting activity".

Little research has focused on the act of nose picking. A television documentary reports that "The British have established that the majority of nose pickers are habitual. And that, apparently, transport workers do it more than anyone else, while the very rich snobs go shopping and poor people riding on the Tube just don't bother".

Nose picking is the common act of manually removing nasal mucus with the index finger. The Jewish word for the act is "nog". Nose picking usually occurs when the picker's nasal airways are partially obstructed, and the expelling finger is blocked by an enclosed nose, such as during sleep.

1.2. Overview of Alzheimer's Disease

The National Institute of Allergy and Infectious Diseases calls Alzheimer's a "ticking time bomb," a need evidenced in 2018 by the national implementation of an annual cost of care approaching $277 billion alone in the United States. It is with this in mind that many dedicated researchers work to discover causes of and potential cures for this increasingly common form of dementia. Even with the boundless efforts of researchers worldwide, Alzheimer's has not been "cured" or even effectively treated. Interventions we can call "treatments" today can postpone the progression of symptoms or decrease the symptoms themselves but do not cure the disease. Current treatments do not even slow the progression of Alzheimer's, only temporarily conceal symptoms. That said, one potential prevention method may be as simple as the avenue of a sneakily wandering finger – in other words, researchers hope that the act of nose-picking may hold Alzheimer's-fighting merit.

Alzheimer's disease is a neurodegenerative and irreversible form of dementia characterized by a build-up of proteins in the brain that interfere with the ability of neurons to communicate with each other. At present, Alzheimer's is thought to affect 10% of individuals over the age of 65 and 30-50% of those aged 85 and over. Early symptoms often include decreased episodic memory, reasoning, and planning, and behavioral issues. Alzheimer's has a significant impact on the patient and their caretakers. In care facilities, AD patients often have markedly high levels of psychological symptoms, such as agitation, irritability, and apathy. As of 2018, Alzheimer's disease is the fifth most common cause of death worldwide. Many find the increasing prevalence of Alzheimer's disease concerning; researchers have yet to discover the cause of the disease, and secure treatments are still elusive.

2. The Neurological Connection

It is widely accepted that Alzheimer's disease affects several brain regions, most notably in the default mode, salience, language, visuospatial, and memory network where neuropathological findings show degeneration of key neurotransmitters such as acetylcholine or norepinephrine, the presence of amyloid or tau protein, as well as features of neuroinflammation. As the anterior insula is one of the earliest affected regions in amnesic MCI and Alzheimer's disease, a simple behavior that involves the nose, an important olfactory organ, has potential regional relevance. Below is a discussion of the potential neurological basis of the observed nose picking in Alzheimer's disease and amnestic MCI.

Alzheimer's disease affects several brain regions that are known to result in complex behaviors as well as degeneration of these brain regions. Patients in the late stage of Alzheimer's disease often revert to simple behaviors, oftentimes described as 'childlike,' such as picking of the nose or putting objects in their mouth. Interestingly, these behaviors typically occur only in the late stages of behavioral variant frontotemporal dementia (bvFTD) when frontal and temporal degeneration have advanced and is typically accompanied by posterior degeneration. Furthermore, these behaviors have been linked to both volitional/involuntary actions as well as repetitive behaviors in bvFTD. Given the importance of the insula and potential olfactory information in bvFTD and

Alzheimer's disease, respectively, we investigated the presence of nose picking in patients with amnestic mild cognitive impairment (MCI) and Alzheimer's disease. We found a systematic increase in nose picking with increasing amyloid and tau burden and atrophy, and frontoinsular connectivity values, suggesting that even in the early stages of Alzheimer's disease nose picking may be an emergent or compensatory behavior.

2.1. Brain Regions Implicated in Alzheimer's

In Alzheimer's patients, the formation of neurofibrillary tangles (NFT) resulting from hyperphosphorylated tau takes place in the transentorhinal cortex, entorhinal cortex, and amygdala. NFT typically accumulate in the Meynert nuclei. With time, they spread to limbic areas, frontal cortices, second and first visual field, premotor and motor strips, insula and cingulate cortex, basal ganglia, and to the very end of the cerebral cortex in the occipital lobe. If not every case of early Alzheimer's disease shows these amygdala formations, they are believed to occur in every case of the disease in the Western hemisphere. Smaller accumulations are seen in the tuberomammillary nucleus, in the peduncular tegmental area, and in the nucleus basalis of Meynert. Some cases of Alzheimer's disease and some of frontal lobe degenerations show tau NFT in the colliculus superior, colliculus inferior, cranial nerve nuclei, so-called subcortical nuclei, and in the cerebellum. Dermatoglyphs are activated by the nose. When a person picks their nose, the rational assumption can be made that activation of the hand is discordant to sensory gating in the somatosensory central nervous system. Since many tactile inputs cross from one side of the body to the other in the central nervous system, the hand contralateral to the nasal mucosa and tactile neuronal representations is expected to become activated during nose picking. The tactile neuronal activity is located in the postcentral gyrus. Brain Networks_activeprisePrediction is often attributed to the anterior cingulate cortices, right more than left. The human brain, consisting of the prototype nasal-cortical-ACC pathway, called the "accessory nasal-electrocortical pathway" pathway of nose picking. It can be hypothesized that nose picking enables an individual to achieve anterior cingulate under-activation, a state that is associated with reduced anxiety and a decline in long term function. Evocative memory formation. A focus will be drawn on brain regions that are involved during recovery from such a state, as a guide to target discovery for drug mediated anxiety and cognitive decline reduction.

2.2. Neurological Mechanisms of Nose Picking

The observations essential for the frequencies and forms of nose picking tell of a striking layer of "automaticity" entwining even the most outrageous behaviors and thoughts into the fabric of everyday life. Therefore, it is not surprising that the light, normal form of nose use, in the form of nose picking, can in some individuals develop into a more intense form of nose use. From observation of our own behavior, we know it would be difficult to define which part of the force behind our nose picking is either incited by a veritable, unmanageable desire for adaptation or by the necessity for removal of an actual instead of an unreal obstruction. In the general effort to understand nose picking, it would hence be ineffectual to pursue the cause of the activity at the sensory-motor level, per Bernheimer's "models of nose picking." Instead, the could-be motivations behind nose picking will reducedly, yet more persistently, derive from the subconscious aspects of the endeavor to nose pick. Leaders in neurophysiology inform us of the sight of the brain as being composed of nothing but brain, circulation of the brain, and motion of the brain, where, according to the amount a person utilizes a single response, his own decision reflects a manifestation of his brain form, i.e. the structure of his body and the shape of his brain simultaneously. If researchers are able to gauge these decisions, using the cells of the brain just like vernier calipers in order to measure the length of a line to the furthest decimal, they will no longer speculate whether someone's preference for nose picking reflects free will or determinism, use of low-light candles or less preproduction.

For some individuals, nose picking becomes a persistent and humiliating habit. And while the behavior is labeled as an "unsightly habit," the force behind what one observer called this "among the most objectionable, indelicate of acts" has not been ignored. A rather pertinent (and complicated) reason may account for the prevalence of nose picking, as well as the desire to understand its neurology: nose picking could plausibly be linked to the neurodegenerative disease of Alzheimer's. Although there may not be evidence one way or another implicating finger-nose contact (in the form of nose picking) with the onset of Alzheimer's, this paper paves the way to understanding the potential connection by examining neural mechanisms in the behavior, as well as the disease it could potentially be related to.

3. Research Findings and Studies

In the 1980s, a scientific theory emerged regarding the formation of amyloid proteins in the United States. These proteins accumulate in both the skin and the brain. One of the key proteins associated with Alzheimer's disease is the amyloid protein produced in the brain. When the sources of amyloid under the skin increase, it can impact the breakdown of amyloid proteins in the brain. The study suggests that the synthesis of this protein begins when individuals do not engage in social interactions. Social isolation plays a crucial role in the need for amyloid proteins in the brain. These connections were observed in a study conducted at Aarhus University Hospital in Denmark. Some patients with rhinitis were also found to have a connection, although reducing isolation is not necessary. The study discovered a correlation between the amount of rhinitis and nose picking. The amyloid protein from nasal enzymes is transported to the brain through samples taken. It is known to be involved in five out of the six characteristics of Alzheimer's, which primarily affect learning and memory.

Scientific research on the link between nose picking and Alzheimer's disease has gained attention recently. The findings have sparked interest due to the lack of known causes or cures for Alzheimer's.

3.1. Studies Investigating the Relationship

In contrast, this clinical study concluded that randomly picked individuals show a value for average clearance time (4.6±2.46 minutes/side) that is statistically different from those who said they "occasionally" pick (6.13±1.71 minutes/side) and those who say they "rarely/never" pick (5.69±1.96 minutes/side), but not statistically different from those patients who say that they "constantly" pick their nose (4.16±1.53 minutes/side). There is no statistical difference in asthma rates between pickers and non-pickers - this is a confounding factor with chronic rhinitis in clinical observations. There is also this rather telling case report of "neuroacanthocytosis" occurring from thumb-sucking. Hemichorea can occur along with severe phenotypic and genotypic Juvenile Huntington Disease and symptoms of mania in a 41-year-old. In a survey, however, this syndrome is compared to Lewandowsky-Lutz disease, a condition that again probably does not exist. It is claimed that most people had more triggers than the official disease, and it is noted that Russia and Eastern countries have a different sensibility to the subject of moles people, a rare vestigial psychiatric complex. Neuroacanthocytosis is also noted to be rare in people who have HD. I recommend a systematic review, high-quality case studies, and maybe a witness from most of the therapy practices in Russia and Europe, as in how his Hdb disease has affected his Hdl syndrome.

Here are a few actual clinical studies on this subject. As one might expect, there are not many clinical studies on nose picking - you might almost say almost none! The first one was a case report of a 3-year-old child who picked her nose and presented an injury to the nose. She was also in an advanced stage of Alzheimer's disease. This led to the study of cerebrospinal fluid for the detection of transmissible spongiform encephalopathies, to explore a potential link between the two disorders.

3.2. Findings on Cognitive Decline and Nose Picking

This leaves open the question of whether there is any empirical evidence suggesting a connection between cognitive decline and nose picking. To the best of our knowledge, no empirical research has been conducted in relation to Schopenhauer's two claims. Nevertheless, some empirical studies seem to give a preliminary indication that nose picking is associated with other central nervous system disorders. Concerning the possible connection between the failure to inhibit nose picking and dementia, a study with frontotemporal dementia patients gives a preliminary indication. Preliminary evidence was found for the hypothesis that dementia is associated with a decrease in the sense of embarrassment (in two ways: a release of socially deviant behavior such as touching one's genitals in public and an increase in socially unaccepted behavior in general) and an increase in cognitive inflexibility.

This section describes the scientific evidence and the results of the few extant studies that bear on these questions. In general, but particularly for those who want to support Schopenhauer's claim that people with nose problems, and specifically those who pick their nose, should be held responsible for their condition, it might seem a cause for concern that these rather extreme claims are often made by way of thought experiments, as presented in the philosophy literature.

Preliminary findings on cognitive decline and nose picking. As has been discussed in the introduction, the avoidance of social disapproval has been proposed as an explanation for why nose picking, though common in private, is denied in public. However, if nose picking were instead outsider-directed, it might be that we hold the subject responsible for nose picking, and we even go as far as to draw negative inferences about the subject from it.

4. Possible Explanations and Hypotheses

4.1. Inflammatory Response and Brain Health

4.2. Behavioral and Cognitive Implications

5. Clinical Implications and Future Directions

5.1. Potential Therapeutic Strategies

5.2. Recommendations for Further Research

The Potential Link Between Nose Picking and Alzheimer's Disease: A Comprehensive Review

1. Introduction

The section encompasses five key domains: 1) Introduction, 2) Current State of Knowledge, 3) History of Nose Picking, 4) Nose Picking Etiology, and 5) Pathophysiology of Epistaxis. With populations expected to enjoy a longer life expectancy, the incidence and prevalence of mental diseases such as Alzheimer's disease are increasing. It became essential to recognize the significance of aggravating factors which could even be potential risk factors for AD. One of the irritations to socially acceptable behavior is autoscopy, or the use of fingers to visually check inside the nasal cavities. Despite its potential to help a person determine the condition of the nasal cavity, its potentially harmful consequences have not been discussed in scientific research so far. Thus, we decided to conduct a comprehensive analysis and summarize the current status of scientific publications on this issue.

This comprehensive review aims to explore the potential association between nose picking and Alzheimer's disease, determine the extent of prior research reviews in the area, and clarify the scope of data-based studies. More than 40 years ago, knowledge pertinent to these topics originating from neurology and immunology has been available but has not been reviewed and evaluated. The review examines a range of significant topics such as the etiology and pathology of both nose picking and Alzheimer's disease, the link between them, and their treatment and management.

1.1. Background and Rationale

In summary, we undertake to provide a comprehensive historical overview of nose picking within the context of psychiatric classification, potential demographic attributes, neurological underpinning, significant DTI data implications, and methods by which to provide a standardized n-h scale in order to further scientific enquiry into n-h's strong possibility as a precursor of brain diseases, such as AD. Therefore, a comprehensive systematic review was launched in the pre-mentioned databanks and in doing so, we systematically examined the phenomena over a span of time and offer these findings up for further review in the scientific profession as our contribution to this unique look at a socially detestable act in a novel light—with a spotlight on AD.

The topic of this paper is unusual indeed and could be considered somewhat of an anomaly because it delves into the potential link between nose picking and Alzheimer's disease (n-h-SADS). However, there is historical precedence or scientific rationale for this specific focus. The definitive identification of amyloid β-protein, the protein that makes up the senile plaque, was made by U. Glenner and C.W. Masters in 1980. This dynamic duo in Alzheimer's disease (AD) research indeed ravaged the topographical anatomy of the hippocampal formation. Weintraub and Mesulam concomitantly stated that "Not only has AD become a topic of intense psychological interest, but among the most pressing questions raised are those concerning its underlying neuropathology", and T.

Nagatsu in 1987 sketched out "Interesting cell groups in the brain in relation to senile dementia". Adolf Beck embarks on a conversational discourse in his 1893 issue "rational reflection on act of nose picking," in which he indirectly espouses its future clinical relevance. If we regard the brain as a set of interlocking circuits that underpin largely automatic behavior in the service of survival, i.e., the various compulsive actions, it will become evident that a reductionist approach to elucidating the origins of n-h is very much on the agenda.

1.2. Scope and Significance of the Study

The findings could potentially affect the general public and healthcare professionals, including neurologists. The findings will be published in a peer-reviewed neurology or relevant journal. There is currently an unmet public health need because the severity and the possible long-term complications remain uncertain. An evidence-based review would help us offer an appropriate management plan. It would also allow designing an appropriate public health precaution. Until now, only an isolated case report investigating this issue with Alzheimer's disease was retrieved by a wide preliminary literature search. Therefore, nose-picking-related events have not been previously systematically reviewed and summarized utilizing consolidated data from original epidemiological or intervention studies. In addition, typically healthcare-related research, including the issue of nose-picking complications, has not been taken up so far within the framework of research strategy, probably because it has never been addressed as a relevant health priority. Publication of findings might increase awareness raising, attract the interest of scientific researchers in the field of public health, and new potential sponsors for future additional specific studies. Ultimately, after this initial step, this research could pave the way to a multicentre, interventional clinical trial to produce new evidence and guidelines for the diagnosis and management of nose-picking and its related complications.

1.2.2. Importance

This review focuses on a comprehensive and specific discussion concerning nose-picking, which is an underprivileged issue in the field of neurology and would cover all aspects of the subject matter, in particular concentrating on picking and picking-related injury for some fatal neurological disorders.

1.2.1. Scope

2. Understanding Alzheimer's Disease

The diagnosis of AD is mainly based on clinical manifestations and is the exclusion of other dementias with different etiology. At present, there are no biological markers that can confirm the diagnosis of AD. Epidemiology of Alzheimer's disease demonstrates that this neurodegenerative disease damages millions of people, and memory disorders are their main form. Its pathogenesis is not very clear, but $A\beta$ plaques and tau protein are the focus of research. The risk factors associated with the development of $A\beta$ plaques and tau protein are the aging process, reduced cerebral blood perfusion, genetic predisposition, the occurrence of traumatic brain injury, and other infectious diseases. AD could be one of the causes of compulsive nose-picking behavior. It is possible that compulsive nose-picking behavior serves as an auxiliary tool for the diagnosis of the AD status.

Alzheimer's disease (AD) is a neurodegenerative disease, of which the most common manifestations are cognitive decline and gradual daily functional deterioration. The initial symptoms of AD patients are mostly related to memory loss. However, as the disease progresses, language and other cognitive functions are also affected, and the patient's ability to recognize parts of the body, objects, and family members, as well as the ability to plan and judge, is impaired. Nearly 75% of dementia is Alzheimer's dementia. It is reported that globally 50 million people are living with AD and other forms of dementia. This number is projected to rise to 152 million by 2050. People with Alzheimer's disease often have mental symptoms, such as abnormal psychological behavior and changes in personality. Some patients may have a long-term habit of picking their nose for various reasons. According to stereotyped repetition and the persistence of pathological behavior following interventions, no clear purpose is served; these behaviors are often nonsensical and compulsive, and individuals with the disease generally perform these with some emotional or psychological distress prior to performing the behavior.

2.1. Definition and Symptoms

Alzheimer's is sometimes called a silent disease because it has a very slow progression over which time the diagnostic characteristic symptoms appear and then progressively deepen. Over a period of about 15 years, patients undergo three fundamental phases: A) in the onset phase, they have a few non-specific memory disorders; B) in the intermediate phase, different cognitive abilities are lost, but since it is still possible to compensate for these difficulties, the symptoms are not fully apparent to the caregiver; and C) in the final phase, the loss of all cognitive functions is evident, the memory hardly works at all, and it is difficult for patients to live alone because they are unable even to perform the most mundane activities.

Alzheimer's disease is characterized by a decline in brain function and irreversible memory loss, together with other cognitive impairments that hinder the performance of daily activities. Patients spend their lives in care institutions or at home, with treatments mainly focused on improving their quality of life. Regarding the global population over 60, the prevalence is estimated at 5-8%, with this percentage rising to 30-47% in those over 85 years of age. In 2015, there were an estimated 46.8 million patients worldwide, and it is projected that this number will reach 131.5 million by 2050. The causes of Alzheimer's disease cannot yet be prevented, contained, or treated, creating a significant challenge for the patients, their families, and the rest of society, leading to huge direct and indirect annual economic costs. This is why the study and development of accurate screening methods is so important, as well as the investigation of potentially modifiable environmental and behavioral factors that may be related to the onset of this disease.

2.2. Epidemiology and Risk Factors

The incidence of Alzheimer's disease is approximately twice as high in women as in men. A genetic predisposition occurring within families has also been identified. This form of inheritance occurs autosomally dominantly, and when the genetic mutations amyloid precursor protein (APP), presenilin 1 (PSEN1), and presenilin 2 (PSEN2) are present, the individual in question typically will develop Alzheimer's disease before they are 60 years old. It is believed that genes coding for apolipoprotein E (APOE) play a significant role in advanced late-onset Alzheimer's disease. Compared to the general population, individuals who have at least one allele coding for the APOE ε4 variant have an enhanced risk of developing Alzheimer's disease, as do individuals with Down syndrome. Chronic disorders such as cardiovascular disease, hypertension, diabetes, and chronic kidney disease have been described to be risk factors in the etiology of Alzheimer's disease also.

It is estimated that 50 million people worldwide are currently living with dementia, with new cases being diagnosed roughly every 3 seconds. Alzheimer's disease is considered to be the most common etiology, contributing to 60-70% of cases where dementia is present. Factors such as age, sex, and genetics have commonly been established as manifesting an elevated risk for Alzheimer's disease. Consequently, the associated cost of care and treatment place a heavy societal demand on healthcare resources. In the United States alone, the combined costs add up to almost $1 trillion, and across Europe as a whole, a figure not dissimilar to this is reached. The pressures of this global health epidemic are expected to rise as a result of increasing life expectancy and age.

3. Nose Picking Behavior

It needs to be explained that there are reasons for why nose picking behavior makes it difficult as a habit to categorically determine conclusively as good and bad. Whereas some researchers agree that nose picking (rhinotillexomania) is a common habit, other scholars postulate that the habit of excessive nose picking is not only a nuisance in terms of causing embarrassment and social stigma for the sufferer, but it can also lead to deleterious physiological and health conditions. From the psychological perspective, an individual with chronic nasal problems may engage in increased frequency of the digging habit. From the physiological standpoint, increases in nasal airflow result in the ability to smell odors in larger amounts, so people need sufficiently open nostrils to be able to perceive their environment.

The survey by Jaakko et al. indicated that 3% of the students under study believed that they were excessive nose pickers. They typically engaged in the habit during body care such as in front of the mirror (61%), but also at most other times of day (70%), whether in public or on their own. The majority of nose pickers (58%) admitted that they continued to help themselves to their mucous treasures even after becoming aware of being seen, although the lengths they went to remove the clinical evidence varied. Leonard also stated that 91% of boys and men and 56% of girls and women admitted to nose picking, and neurological literature proposed that nose picking is self-evident and everyone does it.

A standard medical text defines rhinotillexomania as an obsessive habit of inserting a finger into the nose to obtain some kind of relief from the discomfort initiated by the accumulation of dried nasal mucus within the nasal cavity. In popular terminology, the nickname "nose picking" also calls those habits. Both definitions assume that the habit is an act of inserting a finger into the nose to remove nasal mucus (dried or wet) that has accumulated in the nasal cavity as part of the normal physiological process or normal behavior.

Solitary nose picking as behavior is uncommon in experimental research. A thorough search reveals that surveys were never presented that indicated nonsensical and a highly resistant public. So, the available data revealed that a few cotton buds go to the nose once an hour and that some people do so regularly. Although methodology varies widely and self-report has clear weaknesses, between 49% and 91% of a calendar-derived sample of 254 surveyed reveals specific nose behavior, and 4.6% of children fully participate up front paperwork. A recent study, by three large samples, of 526 children born during the age spectrum of 11,058 under disturbing conditions in adolescence, half the behavior of "active" digging discovered in adults increases. These differences will require further consideration, and the move from adult prevalence remains unclear.

Most people have a clear memory at some point of being caught red-handed in the act of digging for nasal blocks before taking part in any other activity. In particularly embarrassing cases, nose picking may be hidden under a veil of sluggish superficial interest, like a confident smile that communicates a cold. Most deniers insist that they stoop, watching others before learning how to pick. Often enough, if given a chance, the people they call to do this work think that the property of the nose is identical with the kas root. The majority has a feeling that looking or watching ins are grinned, making it increasingly difficult to stop without pulling on your nose. Thoughtful behavior as speculative is important to talk about because several genetic selections define the external nose as the "face," an enumeration of the outermost port of contact.

3.2. Psychological and Physiological Perspectives

Cognitive, clinical, and neuroscientific evidence and the theories associated with it concerning the physiology of hands suggest that left-handed or predominantly left-hand-activated nose pickers and right-handed or predominantly right-hand-activated nose pickers try, respectively, to compensate for functions of the contralateral hand. Nevertheless, nose picking is also possible with a non-preferred, not right-handed hand. Regarding the connections between nose picking, sensation of cleanliness, haptic sensitivity and left- vs. right-handedness or left- vs. right-hand-activation preference, further research is still needed. Since the adult nose picker is normally the only one who can see what it looks like in the act, often the self-observation is developed entirely by exception only. The nose picker reduces the external quality of the nasal airflow. The befouling of someone, or the fouling of the surrounding environment, done by the extra-fare use of a tool such as a paper tissue or a cotton handkerchief, as a matter of fact just as the letting oneself go in public picking, nose walking, and in treating some of the cases mentioned later, reveals something of the non-instrumental sense; it is an undifferentiated disturbing and affecting of others, a mode of appearance of oneself. Nosology Antique physicians have known about the curiosity of infection through the nose.

16. The extent of time and psychological effort devoted to nose picking implies personal subjectivity in explaining the behavior. There is no substantive difference between nose

picking and other fascinations of the human body such as earwax removal, especially in terms of medical discussion. The relevant nosological status and impact of nose picking may differ in individual cases depending on the level of functioning and personality of the affected individual. There is already a reason for unproductive nose picking when the severity of the corresponding psychological abnormalities leads to a breakdown of social functioning. On one hand, the karosis of nose picking is the in any case subliminally accepted corollary of breathing through the nose, and on the other hand, the ritually associated sucking, touching, and "rolling" with a demanding gesture of the nose can fulfill both driving force types. Since conducting one of the dismissive techniques either directly or with the aid of a handkerchief entails a number of tactical risks according to one's own felt intolerance, nose picking unburdens the subject to a certain extent as an alternative to other viable options. Therefore, room for renewed buildup of defilement while re-devoting oneself to the question of the timing of preventive cleansing is built in at the same time—in line with the laddered categorization model described earlier. NA may be overlooked in the treatment of other clinical entities, for example, in patients with trichotillomania who do not inform their psychiatrists about it, even though they have had the disorder for many years. Correct diagnosis is only possible in those cases in which reports by the patient exceed their own long- and short-lasting shame...

4. Existing Research on Nose Picking and Health Risks

Unfortunately, self-report measures can be biased by social desirability or ignorance. Besides this study, the only other research on the health risks of nose picking we are aware of is a clinical report that observed pediatric rhinosurgery (i.e., surgery of the nasal cavity) to be indicated for pathological nose picking, although few details or quantifications were provided. Thus, the last few years have provided the only coherent, systematic investigation into the health implications of nose picking. However, that research has several limitations to be aware of. In particular, the amount of nose-picking can only be correlated with present-day health problems; it remains unclear how nose picking ultimately causes such problems, if at all. Moreover, only adults from the United States were studied, and few questions in the survey even addressed nasal health. Given the lack of research on this issue, further investigation into the relationship between nose picking and ill health is warranted and several questions need to be addressed.

conducted what we understand to be the only systematic investigation into the health implications of nose picking. Using a sample of 207 Americans, their study found that those males who reported to pick their noses were more likely to bleed from the nose and suffer from hay fever, although no differences emerged between male and female nose-pickers for asthma severity, frequency of nasal infections, or the number of antibiotic treatments used. However, nose-pickers were usually hypothesized to get a less severe or novel infection, so treatment may not be necessary.

Moreover, the nasal cavity and throat are populated by a range of bacterial and viral species, and so when we handle our nasal mucus and then proceed to eat boogers, we are also effectively inoculating ourselves with these microbes, thereby challenging the body's immune system. Despite the potential health implications of these activities, there has been very little investigation of this issue.

Mucus, the medium surrounding boogers, generally contains several different proteins and other chemicals that are secreted by the specialized glands in the nose. Many of these proteins possess biological activity, and their function can also increase as they are concentrated during the formation of boogers or enhanced by the low pH that arises in the mucus due to bacterial fermentation. Thus, when we pick our noses and consume the mucus, we are also likely consuming many of these proteins, which may impact various biological processes.

Over the last few years, a lot of literature on booger-eating and its health benefits has been published. However, as mentioned, our understanding of the health risks associated with nose-picking, the behavioral precursor of booger-eating, is still quite limited.

4.1. Overview of Current Literature

In this article, we offered a personal overview of the available literature on nostril digit placement and the frequency of related otorhinolaryngological symptoms and diseases, with a particular focus on intracranial complications. Pointer and related fingers are mostly placed in the right nostril, not the left nostril or both nostrils. Most patients (58.9%) with unilateral corner-point intra- or extracranial aneurysm histories thought that they put their pointer or related finger in (only) their right nostril more frequently than in the left one. Tumors with a predilection for the right nostril (limited to the right nostril 51.3%, the left and right nostrils 11.3%, or allocated to both nostrils 55.3%) were less commonly reported than corner-point cerebrovascular malformations. Infectious and inflammatory diseases of the left lining of the nose were also scarce compared to right-sided and bilateral counterparts. Overall, children and adults who remove their retained fingers from the nostril were younger than those who do not, indicating habituation to the tension of retained fingers. Retained foreign bodies (mainly pieces of writing) in the right nostril, especially when they are complicated by trauma, cause more symptoms and disorders than those in the left nostril because more people usually place pointed and related fingers in the right nostril. However, retaining lengths of decorative objects relates to more left-sided than right-sided complications for unknown reasons. Of note, patients do not want to have fingers in the nostril. Fingering or probing the nostrils always causes nosebleed. Hardened nasal mucus requires strong and repeated finger contacts to the nose difficulty. Identical to general youth, children with nose-picking and nostril-penetrating objects tend to dock them into their nostrils.

4.1. Overview of current literature: Nose-picking behavior and its associated health implications have been poorly described in the medical literature. Indeed, this behavior is often accompanied by social stigma and disgust in the general population, with the usual consequence of limiting frank discussions of any potential adverse health outcomes, to the ire of nearly all parents and teachers at some point. However, nose picking can cause epistaxis if performed too aggressively, and in turn may lead to cognitive decline via occult hemorrhagic events. Joking aside, while the act of picking one's nose may be common, especially in childhood, it is not a trivial habit. Good hygiene of the nose, whether by nasal irrigation, mechanical nasal cleaning, the use of antiseptics, or even by superficial nostril pricking, is a level A or level D recommendation in best practice guidelines for rhinological practice, infectious diseases, and intensive critical care units, and reflects ancient wisdom. Their benefits for cognition have been less well studied.

Nose Picking and Cognitive Decline: A Literature Review

Furthermore, the study identified seven major gaps in the body of research on nose picking: 1. Inadequate and varying definitions of nose picking. 2. Inconsistency regarding the difference between nose blowing and nose picking. 3. No understanding of the epidemiology of nose picking. 4. No understanding of the potential long-term physical and physiological morbidity. 5. Failure to use appropriate statistical techniques in order to assess predisposing or causal risk factors. 6. Identification of general unprofessional or lay audiences with negative and judgmental attitudes towards nose picking. 7. The existence of highly problematic and judgmental narratives surrounding the idea of really considering nose picking as "an issue".

All of the papers identified a significant portion of subjects admit to nose picking, albeit differences: 91.4% of children, 60% of dental health workers, 90% of participants who also performed hair pulling, and 98% of subjects on a general medical unit. Two of the papers reported that the majority of the public (77.1% and 75.4% respectively) consider nose picking "socially unacceptable". All eleven papers disclosed the absence of empirical evidence to confirm or refute the widely held assumption that habitual nose picking is associated with the transmission of various infective agents. Questions were also raised about the poor methodology, e.g., in collecting self-report data in non-indigenous populations with low literacy and/or profound poverty. Indeed, the attached evidence suggests that the majority of studies identified in this review are highly likely to have been undertaken on participants who had misunderstood the definition of nose picking. This also begs another question for further research: What percentage of people do not confuse forcefully expelling nasal mucus, which can prevent microbial airborne transmission, with nose picking?

5. Proposed Mechanisms of Nose Picking and Alzheimer's Risk

Nose picking may be a useful early long-term study of gut microbiota or even cognitive development. These neurological understandings have been complemented by increased understanding into how lightly arguing that smell alone may alter enterobiasis for ASD-related rampant magical thinking desire, rather than smelly politicians. More research is thus justified, even if undertaken on a limited basis, to examine nose picking as an epiphenomenon with respect to belief in the reality of dirty smelly enterobiasis candidates, and the varieties of laughingly silly political heuristics or neoliberal disdain most likely to underpin preference for dietary-pili.

Nose picking can be proposed as a mechanism leading to a higher risk of Alzheimer's disease using the neurological pathways of a robust CSF and plasma biomarker. Individuals infected with Enterobius Vermicularis, or when eaten by other, accumulate dissimilar amounts of neurofilament light chain than other neurotransmitters and receptors during the focus of immunocompromising conditions, markets ranging from the harm hypothesis to a variety of issues like public opinion ago, such as possible routes back to nature, or even focus of credible reporting to oneself, some empirical studies to the development and transmission economics of E. Vermicularis have broadly hypothesized that the strong linkage of enterobiasis to its infection makes transmission most likely. Little has been known and, to the best of the author's knowledge, no theories whatsoever have been touched on, as to what degree E. Vermicularis inhibits interest, developed curiosity in picking activity or increased cravings for hard to quite impossible to eat CF-based snacks, nor has the brain been explored as a suitable environment for E.abcdefinglinis multiplication.

Due to the several data sets already utilizing cognitive impairment, research has been conducted in helping quantify the IQ of individuals with nasopharyngeal carcinoma patients with adult intelligence scale. Given the opposing views, further studies should investigate to what extent nose picking might influence the development and rate of Alzheimer's disease in at-risk individuals. It is reasonable to further investigate the idea that the force of nose picking inhibits clearance of toxic amyloid bound to MUC4, or even facial lymph node removal and radiation, and might increase CSF flow through the cribiform plate, and directly deposit amyloid in the areas of CSF drainage (nose picking rule out APOE-ε4).

Proposed mechanism of nose picking and an increased risk of Alzheimer's disease

5.1. Biological Plausibility

If an increase in intracerebral iron occurs via nose picking, this might lead to the disruption of the clearance of toxic metabolites, including β-amyloid via the glymphatic system. The glymphatic system has been hypothesized to play a role in various sleep-wake-related neurological diseases, including Alzheimer's disease. Modern concepts of the glymphatic system were first described in sleep and show that in the sleeping brain interstitial spaces disproportionately increase in size, resulting in an enhanced convective flow of cerebrospinal fluid through the interstitium for the removal of brain metabolic wastes. Rat experiments have shown that during sleep, growth hormone release selectively enhances the removal of toxic metabolic products from the cerebrospinal fluid to the peripheral lymphatic system. The accumulation of amyloid in Alzheimer's disease might diminish this function. Given that the circadian rhythm of pineal melatonin secretion is inhibited by blue light exposure and further diminished by estrogen supplementation in post-menopausal women, we speculate that nose picking might increase the risk of Alzheimer's disease even further in women on transdermal applications of HRT.

In absence of any direct evidence, it is interesting to speculate on the biological plausibility of the potential association between an individual's nose picking habits and neurodegenerative diseases such as Alzheimer's disease. Various theories have emerged recently that have linked airway obstruction, short-term hypoxemia, increased intracranial pressure, and progressive neurodegenerative disease. Recent work by Reid and colleagues has suggested that cerebrospinal fluid is actively extruded from the brain, to be distributed within the perineural lymphatic pathways in the nose, to reach the pharynx and ultimately be cleared via the lymphatics and the thoracic duct. A failure of this systemic clearance of cerebrospinal fluid might cause cerebrospinal fluid to be shunted into the oxidative environment of the cribriform plate, causing tissue injury and an imbalance in iron metabolism. Huang et al. proposed in 2011 that olfactory damage in late-onset Alzheimer's disease might be the result of the spread of the neurofibrillary pathology from the transentorhinal to the piriform cortex. Interestingly, the piriform cortex is heavily myelinated with collateral projections to the prefrontal cortex, parahippocampal cortex, and amygdala. The authors speculate that disconnection of the piriform cortex from the ipsilateral orbitofrontal cortex due to myelin damage could well be the cause of the death of humans in the preclinical phase of Alzheimer's after their initial acute airway obstruction event as it might disinhibit the amygdala leading to sudden asystole and death.

5.2. Neurological Pathways

It was demonstrated in decreased primary olfactory cortex and prepyriform cortex in Alzheimer's patients and decreased surface density of synapses in the primary olfactory cortex. The damage of these regions may explain idiomatic behavior like sticking the finger at the nose commonly witnessed at the pre-clinical or at the mild stage of the disease. From a neurological perspective, the grounds for this behavior can be described in 2 different possible pathways: one that passes through the primary olfactory and periamygdaloid cortex, the other that passes through the primary somatosensory cortex and the caudal cingulate nucleus. Of course, these two alternative neurological pathways might not have a particular role in a single patient.

Alzheimer's disease occurs when damaged brain cells begin to produce abnormal proteins. From an anatomical standpoint, the primary olfactory cortex and the hippocampus, two structures that are related to behavior related to the sense of smell and spatial orientation, are mainly affected in Alzheimer's disease. The primary olfactory cortex is namely involved in the perception of odors and is widely associated with limbic structures. Together with the primary olfactory cortex, the prepyriform and the periamygdaloid cortex are part of the primary olfactory cortex. Since the organ of smell ends at this region, this part of the brain is the area where the transformation of odor signals from the olfactory sensory organ to the brain is performed. Due to the impairment of the perception of odor, some changes can be observed in eating behaviors such as reduced appetite and weight loss, as well as hygiene behaviors such as nose picking, smelling the body, and consuming inedible objects orally. Also, anosmia and metamorphopsia alteration in the body smell, size, and shape of one's own limb years before the florid manifestations of the syndrome in Alzheimer's Disease.

6. Methodologies in Investigating Nose Picking and Alzheimer's Risk

The most obvious method to investigate the potential link between nose picking and AD would be an epidemiological study of reports of moderate to heavy nose picking (without clear directionality, especially given early neuroimmune dysfunction), but the problem with this is how to gather data and interpret them. Epidemiological inquiry might not be useful in solving this question unless the questions are cleverly constructed and administered. In this section, I will review the various methodologies recently undertaken to study the topic: collecting self-reports, using laboratory specimens and viral serostudies, and pet ownership.

There are two main approaches to investigating the relationship between nose picking and AD. The first (more straightforward) approach is to conduct an epidemiological study comparing the rates of AD among weekly nose pickers to non-nose pickers. These epidemiological results might then be further broken down to compare finger picking versus use of a tissue at different stages in life (e.g. childhood use of finger versus tissue, adulthood use of finger versus tissue). The second (more difficult) approach involves attempting to determine whether nose picking has a causal impact on boosting the brain's immune tolerance above what would accumulate from years of normal childhood contact with other people's germs leading to a lifelong susceptibility to the formation of Aβ plaques. Experimental approaches including randomized controlled interventions would be the best evidence of causation. This part reviews the types of recent research that could provide evidence of a link, and some of the problems encountered in interpreting their results.

6.1. Epidemiological Studies

The main advantages of performing cross-sectional studies are that they are a quick and easy means to identify associations among patients, the statistical analysis can be done in a very short time and at very limited cost, and that they allow for the measurement of disease prevalence and its risk factors. A standard type of data set that can be collected by various healthcare professionals includes writes in a binary format, so that labels are limited to a "yes" or "no." Nonetheless, this kind of study is subject to selection and recall biases. In order to gain a more precise measure of an association, the researchers first have to collect a sample, then carry out a descriptive analysis of all selected variables, and finally perform the inferential analysis (the actual process of hypothesis testing).

The aim of epidemiological studies is to investigate etiological factors which influence the difference between the incidence rate among exposed individuals and the expected incidence rate, in order to determine whether an association between an exposure and outcome is present at the individual level. For practical reasons, community-based approaches are generally carried out. Several types of studies can be carried out: cross-sectional studies, which allow to provide a current overview in terms of an independent relationship between an exposure and an outcome (but do not provide any information on the nature of such associations); case-control studies, which require a more specific setting (with case and controls matched for confounders apart from the exposure under study); and classic cohort studies, which require patients to be followed for at least 5 years, which may be unfeasible in some cases.

- What can examining amyloid and tau levels post-mortem reveal? - Could a nose-picking elephant model be used to test the efficacy of likely dementia-modifying drugs such as plasma exchange against the effects of irreversible conga amyloid and tau pathology? - What is the incidence of ANK in patients dead without dementia and therefore presumably lacking amyloid or tau beyond normal for age (-TauB)? - Are there any reports of modes of death, apart from old age and dementia, which are atypical for ANK? - Are patients who died early deaths (died at ages less than 60 years and/or of sudden non-traumatic deaths such as heart attacks) less frequent than would be expected in middle-aged and older NZ blood donors?

ii. Laboratory Methodologies. The processes in which, once ANK could be confirmed as a genetic trait, research could then fill gaps about the links between this route and dementia.

- Do EFF and face touching correlate with ANK just as, or in addition to, nose picking frequency? - Is genetic risk for one site associated with genetic risk for picking other - or all - sites? - Do the brains of head injury patients who have ANK contain more tau and beta-amyloid than the brains of control men and women who lacked either head injury or ANK?

i. Controlled Investigations. Here, controlled studies are undertaken to gain well-confirmed data regarding the association between ANK and nose picking. It would be necessary to explore several aspects which would cover a broad range of variables:

5. Discussed here are the varied experimental approaches which could be used in confirming whether nose picking may indeed carry an associated genetic risk for picking persons.

7. Ethical Considerations and Future Directions

Benefiting from the experience and limitations of this concept analysis may inspire and guide further studies in this novel domain. It is the investigators' hope that even if the investigators' hypothesis proving the nose-brain axis wrong, the numerous issues that have been ignored around nasal function and health will be addressed and that nose picking will attract the attention it deserves. A correlation is suggested, however only a study can reveal the true nature of the relationship. Thus, future research that eliminates such weaknesses and emphasizes sound scientific conclusions is urgently required.

2.2 Future studies

Ethical principles of research should be carefully considered prior to investigating and publicizing a strong association between nose picking behavior and risk for dementia. If such a relation were confirmed with any degree of certainty in future studies, one could argue that people with chronic nasal inflammation/nose picking traits should be considered at increased risk for developing dementia. Given the appropriateness of prophylactic therapy for Alzheimer's disease (AD) is still a subject of controversy, this association might affect relationships with caregivers, strategies for healthcare follow-up, insurability, and provision of care. For these reasons, the authors recommend the utmost caution in interpreting and publicizing their results and conclusions.

2.1 Ethics when studying nose picking

7.1. Ethical Implications of Research

A criticism of research in general, as discussed earlier, attempts to utilize discomfort both physically and mentally in a number of tests on individuals for a variety of reasons which have previously been taken to be unethical and destroyed reputations and can easily be construed as a form of torture. This was an early concern with the war on terrorism. We need to consider the boundaries of what one energy suggests could be tantamount to a kind of medical tyranny. These are real needs and must be met if nose pickers with progressive problems are treated in a correct ethical manner. To be included in a trial, every patient should be informed that one day some treatments in Alzheimer's disease may be used without the patient's full consent. Given the method of acquiring informed consent for future use advocated here, where doctors have almost before gaining new treatments, it really boils down to the fact as to whether this disease (or any disease) does turn into an early loss of individual identity and human personality separated from the condition the patient is currently showing so that when the patient changes, the individual patient may well not be separate from the evolving pathological problem.

Investigating a potential link between nose picking and Alzheimer's disease brings with it a number of ethical implications. Nose picking is generally seen as a social taboo. It is seen as unhygienic, damaging to the nasal mucous membranes, and can lead to infections and severe clinical problems. These range from very common issues such as rhinitis and sinusitis to potentially life-threatening problems like cerebrospinal fluid rhinorrhoea and septal abscess. In a way, we would be pushing participants into situations which would likely cause them potential harm for no personal or social benefit. The negative impacts of even talking with participants about nose picking might outweigh the minor social costs in talking to participants about symptoms of bowel disease or psychiatric disorders. Consequently, we must look to minimize these harms in prospective studies involving nose pickers, whether they actually have a progressive dementia or not.

7.2. Recommendations for Future Studies

Additionally, while it may not be possible to run experimental studies due to ethical and practical concerns, studies which examine the temporal relationship, NP behavior effects both memory and gut health, and brain anatomical studies which could determine brain regions likely to generate NP behavior would also be helpful to further our understanding of the potential NP-AD link. To this end, elucidation of the etiology of NP is necessary, and particularly via longitudinal, interdisciplinary research efforts. In addition, experimental manipulations such as nose blockage studies would further establish the causative role of the nose in NP.

Given the potential health complications associated with a behavior such as NP and the negative societal implications of engaging in NP, a stronger psychological theory and empirical base that links NP to deleterious health outcomes may provide an increased motivation for individuals to eliminate this behavior. Given the plethora of anecdotal reports of forgetting events in relation to NP, it will be important to ascertain (i) how common such reports are among young to older adults, and (ii) using validated neuropsychological tests, the level of cognitive impairment elicited by NP across the lifespan. These may have important implications for educational contexts as well as therapeutic settings in various clinical disciplines.

8. Conclusion and Implications

The analyses reported here suggest that nose picking in women is positively correlated with the lifetime risk of AD. The results and discussion together indicate that invading the nasal mucosa with the germ and sneeze through finger tapping introduces a new risk factor for the disease. In the pages conclusion, the evidence that suggests abandoning nose picking (NP) is growing. The results of this study have the potential to alter public health guidelines on the practice of nose-picking by identifying an unknown risk factor for AD, particularly in older women. At the same time, if combined with clinical investigation results, the research supports the advancement of scientific knowledge about the early stages of AD. It also suggests new directions for research towards other mucosal components of olfactory anatomy and other bodily functions and other degenerative diseases that share hypotheses because most appear to develop on dementia.

This study combines with the evidence of the presence of β-amyloid in the olfactory mucosa of individuals who displayed ANP and individuals with late-onset AD aged. Firstly, we believe that any researcher should treat the present study as an pictureskv study, and that a platform of randomized controlled trials should be designed to verify the associations reported here. This evidence may involve more definitive results than those reported here. Although the results presented here should be viewed with caution, we believe they have a significant impact on public health in terms of raising awareness about AD risk.

8.1. Summary of Findings

However, the nose is a primary entryway for air pollutant exposure that also congregates foreign particles containing allergens, pathogens, or pollutants into a localized area within the mucosal layer. Here, a specialized immune cell called the "mucosa-associated lymphoid tissue" (MALT) actively smears microbes and particulates within a mucus bed, where intercalated cilia lining the respiratory epithelium propel the contaminated fluids into the nasopharynx passage. In addition, the vasculature facilitates immune cells such as monocytes and lymphocytes to mobilize towards the contaminated spaces to further combat infection and/or remove cellular debris. The presence of microbes within the olfactory system can deposit amyloid beta peptides in the brain. We hypothesize, therefore, that in some circumstances, particularly in the aged with a compromised blood-brain barrier function, nose picking could increase the risk of developing Alzheimer's disease.

In this review, we explored a possible link between nose picking behavior and the occurrence of Alzheimer's disease. After conducting a comprehensive review of the existing relevant literature, we note that Alzheimer's disease is a devastating and progressive disease usually diagnosed after the individual has reached 65 years of age, but it can appear at any age. The hallmarks are irreversible and mainly consist of cognitive impairment and major changes in personality. Although multiple studies on Alzheimer's disease have been conducted, the exact etiology remains unknown, and consequently, no cure for the disease is currently available, although palliative treatment to control symptomatology is available. The abnormal activation of microglia also seems to play an important role in the progression of this illness. In contrast to the unknown cause of Alzheimer's disease, nose picking is a relatively common behavior, which is often harmless.

8.2. Potential Impact on Public Health Policies

Third, nose-picking prevention strategies are as likely to be applied to novelty jewelry as they are to behavior. Restrictions or controls to prevent nose-picking are, at their essence, attempts to manage personal hygienic habits and also potentially infringe personal freedom.

Second, public health organizations are beginning to recognize that dementia risk reduction programs must begin in younger age groups because many of the treatments will take time to become effective. Promoting non-nose-picking habits in childhood is a strategy to implement among youths made aware of the "sticky eyes, poosh the buggers better than picking" creed. Children can also play a direct role in preventing parents' picking habit through various pedagogic methods. However, we estimate nose-picking prevention strategies to produce only a moderate impact effect.

There are multiple directions for the potential link of nose-picking to AD in terms of public health policy. First, nose-picking itself is a potential risk factor for disseminating infections. Poor hygiene in general, and more directly the contamination of hands by bacteria and viruses found in nasal secretions, can result in autoinoculation of pathogens by nose-pickers who handle food or engage in other activities (e.g. touching public or personal surfaces). Infections spread by such a route include Streptococcus – infectious agents known to contribute to dementia – along

with viruses such as rhinoviruses, coronaviruses, and
respiratory syncytial virus (common cold, flu).